YOUR KNOWLEDGE HAS VALUE

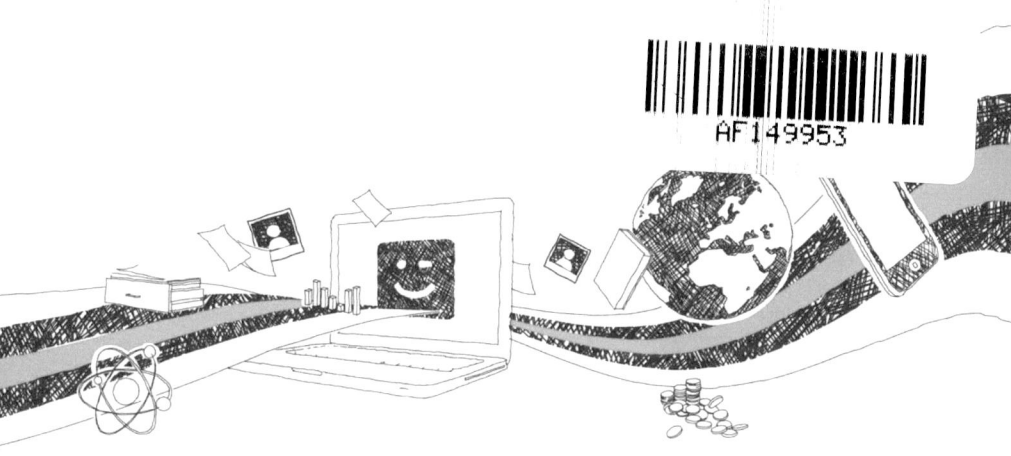

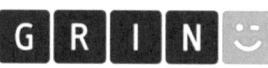

Dr.Sibi P.Ittiyavirah

Hepatoprotective activity of Kamilari

GRIN Publishing

Bibliographic information published by the German National Library:

The German National Library lists this publication in the National Bibliography; detailed bibliographic data are available on the Internet at http://dnb.dnb.de .

Imprint:

Copyright © 2012 GRIN Verlag GmbH
Print and binding: Books on Demand GmbH, Norderstedt Germany
ISBN: 978-3-656-59943-2

This book at GRIN:

http://www.grin.com/en/e-book/268298/hepatoprotective-activity-of-kamilari

GRIN - Your knowledge has value

Since its foundation in 1998, GRIN has specialized in publishing academic texts by students, college teachers and other academics as e-book and printed book. The website www.grin.com is an ideal platform for presenting term papers, final papers, scientific essays, dissertations and specialist books.

Visit us on the internet:

http://www.grin.com/

http://www.facebook.com/grincom

http://www.twitter.com/grin_com

Anti steatosic effects of Polyherbal Formulation 'Kamilari'

*Sibi P.Ittiyavirah, Anjana R.S. and Rahees T.

Department of Pharmacology, University college of pharmacy, Cheruvandoor campus, M.G.University, Kottayam, Kerala, India-686631

ABSTRACT

Polyherbal formulations available with a wide range of indications like hepatoprotective , appetite and growth promoters, gastrointestinal and hepatic regulator, as treatment for hepatic dysfunction, for hepatic regeneration as well as liver stimulant and tonic. Despite the widespread use, there is a lack of scientific evidence on their efficacy and safety. This study was designed to evaluate the effect of Polyherbal formulation Kamialri on oxidative stress and associated damages in carbon tetrachloride induced toxicity in Chang liver cells. The study is mainly focused on the evaluation of its antioxidant potential, *invitro* steatosis and intracellular localisation of reduced glutathione by Monochlorobimane(MCB) staining. Carbon tetrachloride induced toxicity in chang liver cells was well manifested by significant decrease in cell viability, enhanced lipid peroxidation leading to tissue damage,decreased SOD, glutathione, glutathione peroxidase and glutathione S- transferase and increased deposition of fatty acid . MTT study revealed that Kamilari has got cytoprotective activity. It has got the excellent free radical scavenging properties which was proven by various antioxidant activities (LP, SOD, GSH, GPX, GST) . Inhibitory effect of Kamilari on fatty acid deposition was proven by *invitro* steatosis studies which was conducted on palmitic acid treated chang cell line.

Based on the above studies it is concluded that Kamilari has cytoprotective and antioxidant activity, and found to be effective in steatosis .

Keywords : polyherbal formulation, kamilari, steatosis, hepatoprotective activity.

1. Introduction

Liver is an important *organ* that plays an essential role in regulating various physiological processes in the body. It is involved in several vital functions, such as metabolism, secretion and storage. *In vitro* liver systems represent a better experimental approach to screen potential hepatotoxic compounds . Liver cell lines are characterized by unlimited subcultivation and cell availability in large number[1] . The hepatotoxin used was carbon tetrachloride because it has long been known as a model toxicant and has been the focus of many *in vitro* and *in vivo* toxicological studies[2]. The liver is the major target organ of carbon tetra chloride toxicity owing to its high content of Cytochrome P-450[3].

Kamilari is a commercial ayurvedic formulation suggested to be effective in treatment of liver disorder such as **jaundice, chronic alcoholism, acute and chronic inflammatory disorders.** As per the manufactures information Kamilari consist of *Thespesia populinea, Eletteria cardamom, Zingiber officinalis, Glyccyrhiza glabra, Piper longum, Aegle marmelos, Trichosanthes cucumerina, Holostemma adakodein Schulter* and *Honey.*Since large mass of populations used preferable herbal preparation, therefore there is need to be evaluate the proper mechanism underlying the hepatoprotective effect.

Kamilari, a polyherbalformulation of traditional medicinal plants and its *in vivo* protective effect being reported[4] but no valid data is available regarding proper cellular mechanism on carbon tetrachloride toxicity . **This study was designed to evaluate the effect of Kamialri on oxidative stress and associated damages in Ccl₄ induced toxicity in Chang liver cells.** The study is mainly focused on the evaluation of its antioxidant potential, *invitro* steatosis and intracellular localisation of reduced glutathione by Monochlorobimane(MCB) staining.

2. MATERIALS & METHODS

2.1 Invitro protective effect of Kamilari in Ccl₄ treated Chang liver cells

Chemicals and media.

Carbon tetrachloride(0.1%) (Appendix 1), Trypsin (Appendix 1), Foetal bovine serum albumin (Appendix 1), Palmiticacid(20Mm) (Appendix 1), Oil red O (Appendix 1), MTT (3-(4, 5-dimethylthiazolyl)-2, 5-diphenyl-tetrazolium bromide) (Appendix 1),Dimethyl sulfoxide (Appendix1) .

MTT assay[5].

500µl Dimethyl Sulphoxide (DMSO) , Chang liver cell line, Micropipette, Medium –DMEM with 10% FBS pH 7.4, 500µl MTT in PBS, CO2 incubator, UV-Visible spectrophotometer

2.2 Lipid peroxidation[6]

70% alcohol,1%TBA,400µl acetone,Cell lysate

2.3 Estimation of SOD activity[7]

50mM phosphate buffer (7.8), 45µM methionine, 5.3mM riboflavin, 84µM NBT, 20 µM potassium cyanide, cell lysate(50µl).

2.4 Estimation of reduced glutathione[8]
1ml of cell lysate., 0.5 ml of phosphate buffer (0.2M pH 8), 1.3 ml of distilled water ,0.2 ml of DTNB (0.6mM).

2.5 Assay of Glutathione peroxidase[9]
2ml phosphate buffer (0.1 M, pH 7.4), 0.3 ml of 20 mM sodium azide, 0.2 ml (15mM EDTA), 0.1ml (1mM GSH), 0.1ml (0.1mM NADPH), 0.5 ml water.

2.6 Glutathione -s-transferase[10]
100mlpotassium phosphate buffer pH 6.5, 1mM EDTA,1mM,1 chloro2,9dinitrobenzene(CDNB),1mM reduced glutathione

2.7 Oil Red O [11](Spectrophotometric method)
Kamilari,Palmitic acid, Phosphate buffered saline, Oil red O, Isopropanol
Monochlorobimane(MCB)FlourescentStaining

Kamilari,MCB,PBS

Culturing and maintenance of *Chang liver cells*
Chang liver cells were purchased from National centre for cell science,Pune and maintained in Dulbecco's Modified Eagles Medium (DMEM) containing L-glutamine with high glucose

Cell culture and treatment
Chang liver cells were cultured in DMEM medium supplemented with 20% heat inactivated foetal bovine serum. Antibiotics (Streptomycin and Penicillin) was added to prevent bacterial contamination. The culture was filtered and sterilized using 0.2μm pore size cellulose acetate filter.
Chang liver cells was used for *invitro* evaluation of the possible hepatoprotective activity of Kamilari. Foetal bovine serum albumin was used to provide sufficient amount of nutrients for the proper growth of chang cell line. The cell line were washed with phosphate buffer saline and the fully confluent cells were trypsinised using 500μl of trypsin for 3 min at 37^0C. After disaggregation, the cells were transferred to other flask and supplemented with media.

Hepatoprotective effect of kamilari on Ccl4 induced toxicity in *Chang liver cells*.
Ccl4 was used to induce hepatotoxicity on change liver cell line. The cytoprotective effect of kamilari in Ccl4 treated chang liver cells were determined by assessing the viability and intracellular antioxidants. Ccl4 was added to a final concentration of 0.1% followed by different concentration of polyherbal formulation such as 5 and 10μl. Silybon70μg/ml was used as standard and an untreated flask was maintained as negative control. All experiments were carried out triplicate and proved to be statistically significant.

1. **Cytoprotective effect of Kamilari in chang liver cells**

MTT ASSAY[5]

MTT is a colorimetric assay that measures the reduction of yellow 3(4,5 dimethythiazol-2-yl)-2, 5-diphenyl tetrazolium bromide (MTT) by mitochondrial succinate dehydrogenase.

Effect of Kamilari on Ccl₄ induced oxidative damage.

Cell lysis

The treated cells were scrapped and collected from tissue culture flask were lysed using lysis buffer and the cell debris was precipitated by centrifuging at 2000 rpm in 10ml at 4^0C and supernatant was used for assay.

Estimation of lipid peroxidation[6]

Lipid peroxidation is referred as the oxidative degradation of lipids. Polyunsaturated fatty acid peroxides generate malondialdehyde (MDA) upon decomposition, and the measurement of MDA has been used as an indicator of lipid peroxidation.

Estimation of SOD activity[7]

Superoxide dismutase uses the photochemical reduction of riboflavin as oxygen generating system and catalyses the inhibition of nitro blue tetrazolium (NBT) reduction,the extent to which can be assayed spectrophotometrically at 600nm.

Estimation of reduced glutathione[8]

The tripeptide GSH is present in cells at millimolar concentrations. Under normal conditions, most of the GSH is maintained in its reduced form by glutathione reductase. Continual production of reactive oxygen species, such as H_2O_2, OH^-, and lipid peroxides, leads to accumulation of oxidized glutathione (GSSG). A concomitant reduction in the level of GSH provides a relevant and accurate measure of the oxidative state of the cell.

Assay of Glutathione peroxidase[9]
It is based on the oxidation of glutathione (GSH) to oxidized glutathione (GSSG) catalyzed by GPX, which is then coupled to the recycling of GSSG back to GSH utilizing glutathione reductase (GR) and NADPH (Nicotinamide Adenine Dinucleotide Phosphate, reduced). The decrease in NADPH absorbance measured at 340 nm during the oxidation of NADPH to NADP+ is indicative of GPx activity.

Glutathione -s-transferase[10]

The method to assay of GST activity involve measuring the conjugation of 1- chloro-2,4 dintrobenzene(CDNB) with reduced glutathione. The conjugation of GSH with CDNB was read at 340 nm.

Invitro induction of hepatic steatosis by supplementation of Palmitic acid.

Hepatic steatosis, or fatty liver, is characterized by the excessive accumulation of triglycerides in the form of lipid droplets in the liver.

Preparation of Palmitic acid BSA Colloidal Solution

Palmitic acid (25 mM) in 0.01N sodium hydroxide was incubated at 70^0C for 30 min and it was filtered using a sterile filter. 5g palmitic acid in 5ml BSA solution was prepared in double distilled water and filtered using a sterile filter . Fatty acid soaps were then complexed with 5% BSA in PBS at 7:1molar ratio of fatty acid to BSA.

The palmitic acid BSA conjugates were administered to the cultured cells to induce steatosis and it was determined by Oil Red O (Spectrophotometric method) andOil Red O(Microscopic method)

Oil red O (spectrophotometric method)[11]
Oil red O (microscopic method) (Anusha et al.,2006)[11]

Intracellular Localisation of reduced glutathione by Monochlorobimane (MCB) Flourescent Staining[12]

Reduced glutathione shares a considerable role in scavenging oxidative damage of cells providing cell protection. A significant decrease in reduced glutathione can lead the cells to oxidative damage.

2. Statistical analysis

Statistical analysis was performed by using Graph pad prism version 6.0.All the experiments were expressed as mean±SD. Data were analysed using one way ANOVA followed by Post hoc Dunnet multiple comparison test , $P<0.05$ were considered as statistically significant.

3. RESULTS

3.1 Cytoprotective effect of Kamilari in Chang liver cells.

MTT Assay

Chang cells were treated with 0.1% Ccl4 which was experimentally proved to be cytotoxic for checking the cytoprotective activity of Kamilari. The addition of Kamilari increase the cell viability to 69% where as the viability Ccl4 was 40% (Fig.1). The result confirms the amelioration of Ccl4 induced toxicity by Kamilari in a dose dependant manner. . **It was found that Kamilari at 10 µl exhibited a significant (P<0.001) cytoprotective effect** (Fig1).

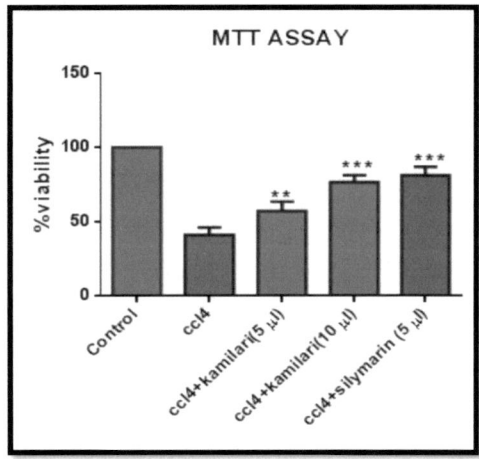

Fig.1 Cytoprotective effect of Kamilari on Ccl4 induced in chang liver cell was determined by the MTT assay one way ANOVA P value<0.001, F-212.5, Df-4

3.2 Antioxidant enzymes and markers

The antioxidant enzymes and markers were assayed on the sample treated chang cells.

Lipid peroxidation

The level of MDA, which is one of the end products of lipid peroxidation in liver cells, was found to be high in Ccl4 group implying enhanced lipid peroxodation leading to tissue damage. Treatment with silymarin significantly reverse this effect (Fig 2). It was found that Kamilari at 5µl exhibited significant (P< 0.05) lipid peroxidation by compared to toxicant group.

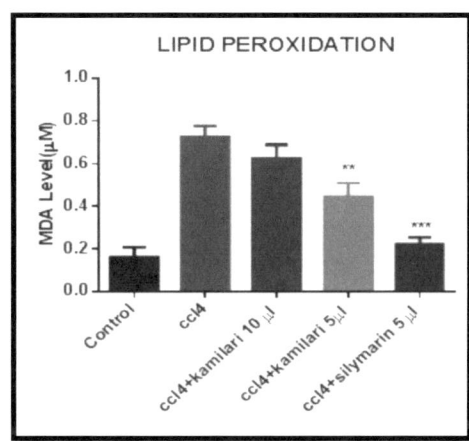

Fig 2: Effect of Kamilari on hepatic lipid peroixidation activity in chang liver cell line.

P value-0.0229, F-146.81, Df-4

Superoxide dismutase (SOD)

Superoxide dismutase is an indicator of cytotoxicity of many free radical generating species. It was found that that Kamilari at 5µl exhibited significant (P<0.001) SOD activity(Fig3)

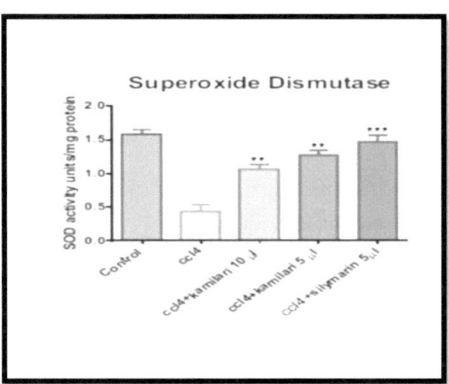

Fig 3: Effect of Kamilari on hepatic super oxide dismutase acticity in chang liver cell line.
P value-0.001, F-311.4, Df-4

Reduced glutathione (GSH)

The GSH was normally increased in the untreated cells, and this level was decreased in the presence of Ccl4. But this effect was reversed by the addition of kamilari 5µl. It was observed that Kamilari at 5µl exhibited a significant (P<0.001) glutathione activity(Fig4).

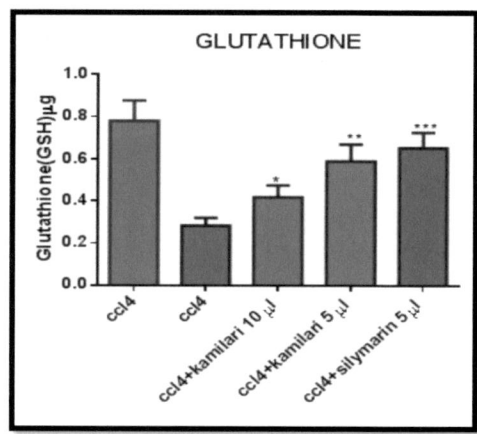

Fig4: Effect of Kamilari on hepatic Glutathione   acticity in chang liver cell line. One way ANOVA **P value-0.001, F-115.48, Df-4**

Glutathione Peroxidase

The Glutathione peroxidase was normally increased in the untreated cells, and this level was decreased in the presence of Ccl4.It was found that Kamilari at **5µl** exhibited a significant (P<0.001) glutathione peroxidase activity (Fig 5)

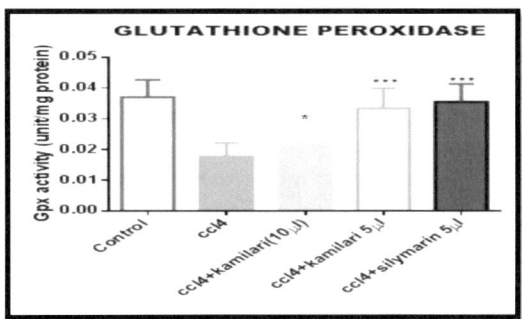

Fig 5: Effect of Kamilari on hepatic Glutathione peroxidase acticity in chang liver cell line.: P value-0.001, F-123.46, Df-4

Glutathione- S-transferase(GST)

It was found that Kamilari at **5µl** exhibited a significant (P<0.001) Glutathione peroxidase activity.

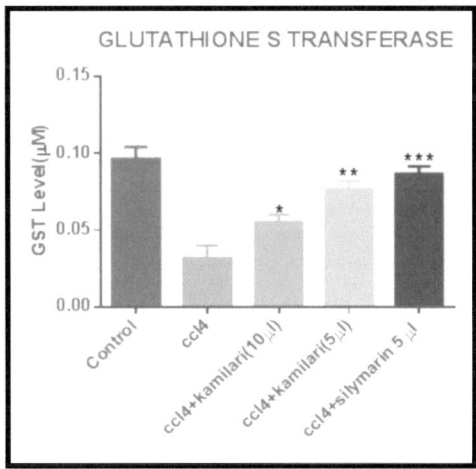

Fig 6 : Effect of Kamilari on hepatic Glutathione transferase acticity in chang liver cell line. One way ANOVA **P value-0.001, F-223.12, Df-4**

Oil red o (Spectrophotometric method)

Steatosis is a pathological disorder characterized by abnormal accumulation of lipids within the cells and this is considered as a significant parameter in evaluating the hepatoprotective effect of the drug .Oil red o stain neutral triglycerides and lipids which was shown spectrophotometrically. It was found that Kamilari treated cells exhibited significant (P<0.05) activity when determined by oil red o spectrophotometrically (Fig 7) .

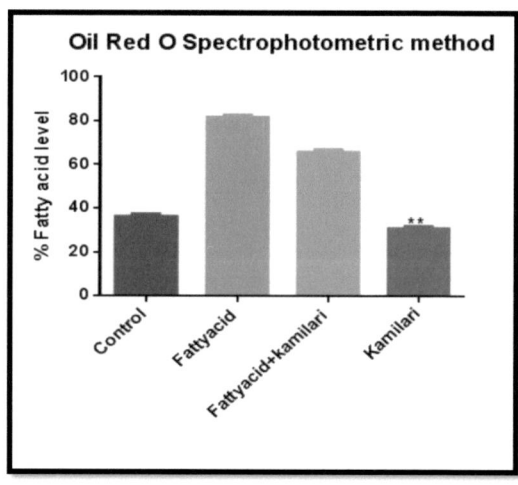

Fig 7: Effect of kamilari on steatosis by Oil red o (Spectrophotometric method) P value-0.0023, F-223.46, Df-3

Oil red o (Microscopic method)

Oil red o stains neutral triglycerides and fats which was observed from microscopical studies. It was found that fatty acid nontreated cells shows no deep red stain where as addition of Palmitic acid BSA suspension increase the intracellular uptake of fatty acid as evident from dark red spots(Fig17). Addition of Kamilari significantly decreased the number of red droplet .

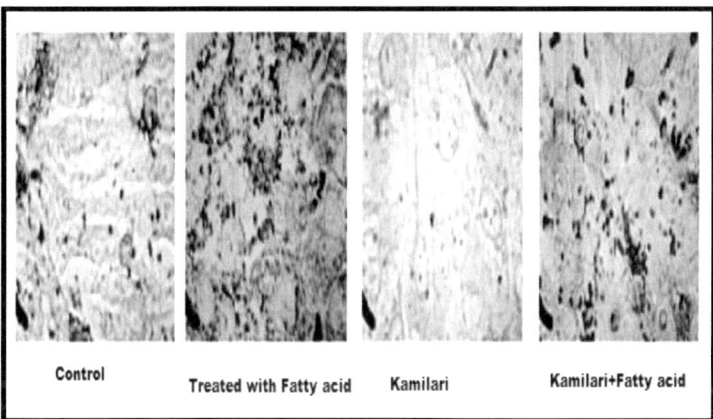

Control   Treated with Fatty acid   Kamilari   Kamilari+Fatty acid

Fig 8: Effect of Kamilari on steatosis by oil red o staining in chang liver cell line by microscopic method. Intracellular lipid accumulation shown by red spots.

Intracellular localisation of reduced glutathione by Monochlorobimane (MCB) **flourescent staining.**It was observed that Ccl_4 treatment significantly decreased glutathione content by decreasing fluorescence. Addition of Kamilari significantly increase in green fluorescence suggesting that decreased oxidative damage to the cells (Fig9).

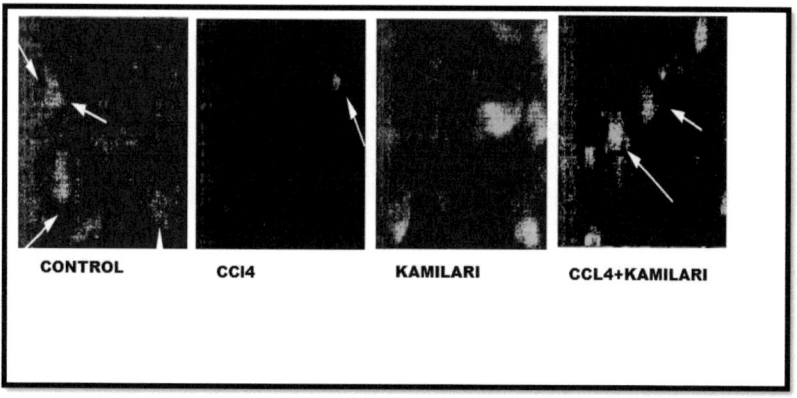

| CONTROL | CCl4 | KAMILARI | CCL4+KAMILARI |

Fig 9: Intracellular localisation of reduced glutathione by Monochlorobimane (MCB) flourescent staining in chang cell line shown by green fluorescence.

4. Discussion

The liver is a vital organ of paramount importance involved in the maintenance of metabolic functions and detoxification of the exogenous and endogenous challenges like xenobiotics, drugs, viral infections and chronic alcoholism[13] (Ramachandra et al., 2007). Recent statistical survey revealed that death toll due to hepatic disorders is increasing in number but there is only limited number of drugs available for the treatment. The virus and reactive oxygen species are the main causes of liver damage, hence an antioxidant may be a useful tool for protecting the liver cells against superoxide anion radicals (O_2 •−), hydrogen peroxide (H_2O_2), hydroxyl radicals (OH•), and the singlet oxygen [O] induced damage[14] (Jain et al., 2008).

Kamilari is an ayurvedic polyherbal formulation claimed to be effective in the treatment of liver disorders such as jaundice, chronic alcoholism, acute and chronic inflammatory disorders. Chang liver cells are non malignant, healthy human liver cells widely used for evaluation of hepatoprotective/hepatotoxic studies[15] Ccl_4 was used for inducing *invitro* hepatotoxicity based on previous references of Suredaran et al .,2011[16].

In our study steatosis was induced by using colloids of Palmitic acid in bovine serum albumin. Kamilari was found to be effective in reducing the amount of accumulated lipid droplets when determined by Oil red O spectroscopy and microscopy(Fig7 and 8). **The result strongly suggest that it is effective in steatosis condition**.

MTT assay revealed that Kamilari has got cytoprotective activity at a conc. of 10μl. It has got the excellent free radical scavenging properties which was proven by various antioxidant activities (LP, SOD, GSH, GPX, GST) and got activity at 5μl. Inhibitory effect of Kamilari on fatty acid deposition was proven by *invitro* steatosis studies which was conducted on Palmitic acid treated chang cell line. By verifying the results of Monochlorobimane (MCB) fluorescent staining studies we can summarized that Kamilari has got excellent capacity to increase the reduced glutathione content in chang cell line.

5. **Conclusion**

The results obtained from the present study revealed that the Kamilari posssesed the cytoprotective effect and antioxidant activity. However the antioxidant effect of Kamilari shows highly effective at **small doses(5μl)** while the effect was reduced at high doses**.** The *invitro* steatosis study confirms the inhibitory effect on Kamilari on fatty acid deposition . Kamilari shows significant increase in reduced glutathione content by MCB staining . Based on the above studies it is concluded that Kamilari is effective in cytoprotecive effect in chang cell line, and shows antioxidant effect and also effective in steatosis .

The investigation of exact mechanisms and more pharmacokinetic studies have to be conducted to evaluate the role of clinical administration of Kamilari in liver disease .More studies are also required to evaluate the mechanism underlying the effect of Kamilari in increasing the efflux of fatty acid and reducing risk of steatosis.

BIBLIOGRAPHY

1. Guillouzo A. Liver cells models in invitro toxicology. Environ Health Perspective. 1998;106: 511- 32.
2. Manibusan MK, Odin M, Eastmond DA. Postulated carbon tetrachloride mode of action : A review. *J Environ Sc Health.* 2007; 25 : 185 -209.
3. Sodergren E, Cederberg J, Vessby B, Basu S. Vitamin E reduces lipid peroxidation in experimental hepatotoxicity in rats. *Europ J Nutrition.* 2001; 40(1) : 10 – 16.
4. Rajesh MG, Latha MS. Preliminary evaluation of the antihepatotoxic of kamilari, a polyherbal formulation. *J Ethnopharm.*2004; 91 : 99 – 104.
5. Arung ET, Britanto DW, Yohana AH, Irawan WK, DinaY, Ferry S. Anticancer properties of diethyl ether extract of wood from Sukun (*Artocarpus altilitis*) in human breast cancer (T47D) cells. *Trop J Pharm Res.* 2009; 8(4) : 317- 324.
6. Ohkawa H, Onishi N, Yagi K. Assay of lipid peroxidation in animal tissue by thiobarbituric acid reaction. *Anal Biochem.*1979; 95 : 351 – 358.
7. Misra HP, Fridovich I. Determination of the level of super oxide dismutase in whole blood. *Yale Univ Press New* Haven.1972; 101 – 109.
8. Moron MS, Depierre JW, Mannervik B. Levels of glutathione, glutathione reductase and glutathione s- transferase activities in rat lung and liver. *Biochem. Biophys.Acta.* 1979; 58 (2):67 - 78.
9. Wendel A. Glutathione peroxidases. In : Enzymatic Basic of Detoxification. *Academic Press, New York.* 1980; 333 – 353.
10. Mannervik B, Alin P, Guthenberg C, Jenson, Tahir H, Arholm MW, Jornvall H. Identification of three classes of cytosolic glutathione transferase common to several mammalian species : correlation between structural data and enzymatic properties. *Int J Exp Biol.* 1985; 82 (21) : 7202-7206.
11. Anusha AA, Ravikumar DR, Cliff JF, WeiL W, Hong YG, Gour MH, Jen LW. Thioacetamide induced liver damage in zebrafish embryo as a disease model for steatohepatitis. *J Biomedical Scienc. B* 2006; 225-232
12. Kamencic H, Lyon A, Paterson PG, Juurlink BH. Monochlorobimane flourometric method to measure tissue glutathione. *Anal Biochem.*2000; 286 : 35 – 37.
13. Ramachandra SS, Absar AQ , Viswanath SA, Tushar P, Prakash T, Prabhu K, Veeran GA. Hepatoprotective activity of calotropis procera flowers against paracetamol – induced hepatic injury in rats. *Fitoterapia.*.2007; 78 : 451 – 454.

14. Jain A, Soni M, Deb L, Jain A, Rout S, Gupta V, Krishna K. Antioxidant and hepatoprotective activity of ethanolic and aqueous extracts of Momordica dioica Roxb. Leaves. *J Ethanopharmacol*.2008; 115(1) : 61-66.

15. Chang RS. Continuous subcultivation of epithelial – like cells from normal human tissues. *Proceedings of the Society for Experimental Biology and Medicine*.1954;87: 440-443.